Primary Care:
Understanding Health Need
and Demand

National Primary Care Research and
Development Centre Series

Primary Care:
Understanding Health Need
and Demand

National Primary Care Research and Development Centre Series

Anne Rogers

and

Heather Elliott

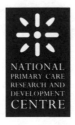

NATIONAL
PRIMARY CARE
RESEARCH AND
DEVELOPMENT
CENTRE

RADCLIFFE MEDICAL PRESS

Radcliffe Medical Press Ltd
18 Marcham Road, Abingdon, Oxon OX14 1AA, UK

Radcliffe Medical Press, Inc.
141 Fifth Avenue, New York, NY 10010, USA

British Library Cataloguing in Publication Data

A catalogue record for this book is available from the British Library.

ISBN 1 85775 237 6

Library of Congress Cataloging-in-Publication Data is available.

Typeset by Advance Typesetting Ltd, Oxon
Printed and bound by Biddles Ltd, Guildford and King's Lynn

The National Primary Care Research and Development Centre is a Department of Health-funded initiative, based at the University of Manchester. The NPCRDC is a multi-disciplinary centre which aims to promote high-quality and cost-effective primary care by delivering high-quality research, disseminating research findings and promoting service development based upon sound evidence. The Centre has staff based at three collaborating sites: The National Centre at the University of Manchester, The Public Health Research and Resource Centre at the University of Salford and the Centre for Health Economics at the University of York.

For further information about the Centre or a copy of our research prospectus please contact

Maria Cairney
Communications Officer, NPCRDC
The University of Manchester
5th Floor, Williamson Building
Oxford Road
Manchester M13 9PL

Tel: 0161 275 7633/7601

Contents

About the authors

Anne Rogers is a Senior Research Fellow at the National Primary Care Research and Development Centre (NPCRDC) and Reader in Sociology at the University of Manchester. She is also a Programme Area Leader for Population Health and Demand for Care at NPCRDC.

Heather Elliott is a NPCRDC Research Fellow based at the University of Salford's Public Health Research and Resource Centre.

Acknowledgements

This briefing paper draws on a number of working papers and a number of my colleagues at the National Primary Care Research and Development Centre have been consulted during the preparation of these. I am grateful for their helpful advice, editing, comments and for providing literature and ideas which have informed the analysis presented here. These colleagues include Helen Busby, Tom Butler, Caroline Glendinning, Gerry Nicolaas, Jennie Popay and Martin Roland.

I am indebted to Bernice Pescosolido of Indiana University for providing me with her collected works on health care utilization and to David Pencheon for his working paper *On Demand.*

Thanks are also due to David Pilgrim and Stephanie Short for their thoughtful comments and sociological insights.

Finally, I am grateful to Eileen Rendall for her secretarial support and help with references.

Anne Rogers
April 1997

1

Introduction

This book provides a summary analysis of the clinical, sociological, policy and other literature relevant to understanding the key factors shaping the relationship between health need, demand and health care utilization. A wide range of literature from the disciplines represented in health services research has been covered in the work informing this analysis. In addition to empirical findings, key policy and conceptual issues relevant to need and demand for primary care services are represented. The analysis presented here was set in the context of work being undertaken in the National Primary Care Research and Development Centre's (NPCRDC) programme on Population Health Need and Demand for Primary Care.

The main aim of early research work in this programme area has been to identify the factors shaping the relationship between demand for, and use of, primary care. This aim involves an examination of the patterns and social processes influencing the use of formal primary care and the relationship between people's conceptions and experience of illness, self- and informal management of illness and their use of formal services. This analysis is orientated towards providing a detailed picture with which to inform the planning of appropriate, acceptable and responsive primary care services. An understanding of lay decision-making in the use of formal services is important in relation to current primary care service debates about 'the management of demand', patient responsibilities and the role of self- and mutual care that patients contribute to primary care provision.

THE SCOPE OF THE STUDY

The summary provided here presents the main messages and picture gleaned from carrying out searches on numerous databases and the scrutiny of abstracts, articles and key texts. There are both population and supply factors which impinge on patient demand for, and use of, primary care services. The main focus has been placed on the former but recognition is also given to supply and service factors. The intention has not been to provide a comprehensive review of all the pertinent literature of the findings in these areas. Rather, the aim has been to review selected studies which identify the range of factors which influence people's use of services, and to highlight limitations of work to date. The latter implies and points up approaches which have potential for better understanding of contemporary need, demand and use of services. As such, the study is a critical review.

Literature reporting or exploring concepts and empirical findings are organized in this book under the following headings:

* Patient need, demand and use of primary care
* Perspectives in the study of service utilization
* Help-seeking and health care as a social process
* The relevance of lay concepts and experience of illness for help-seeking
* The relevance of social networks to help-seeking
* Individual self-care and lay care provided by others

- Organizational factors influencing demand for, and use of, services
- The influence of information on patient decision-making.

Defining primary care

The definition of primary care adopted in this review is one which views primary care as the *utilization* of the various sources of care available to respond to new illness episodes. This includes the less visible self- and informal primary care provided by non-professionals. From this perspective, patients are not seen simply as the recipients of care but also as providers or co-providers of primary care. This varies from more traditional definitions of primary care as constituted by the *organizational* aspects of formal service provision, which includes general practice and primary health care teams with pharmacy and other practitioners operating at the periphery.

2

Patient need, demand
and use of primary care

There are few presumptions in human relations more dangerous than the idea that one knows what another human being needs better than they do themselves.[1]

Needs have to be felt as such, perceived, then expressed in demand.[2]

THE POLICY CONTEXT OF NEED AND DEMAND

Studies on utilization carried out in the 1960s and 1970s were concerned with under-utilization and unmet need.[3,4] More recently there has been a greater concern with 'inappropriate' demand, though, interestingly, both generations of research tend to view patient behaviour as the focus of the problem. Definitions of need and demand used in the literature vary across time and according to lay, policy and professional perspectives.

The review also highlights the coexistence of different interests in the process of defining needs and demand for care. Of particular relevance to primary care health services' research is the observation that different concepts of need coexist within National Health Service (NHS) policy-making.[5] The most commonly deployed concept of health care need in current health care policy is orientated towards the maintenance of existing health service practice and priorities and clinical and cost-effectiveness. From this perspective, the 'management of demand' tends to be viewed as a clinical problem for which there is an effective health care intervention.[6,7] In contrast to this, social science literature has emphasized the relative and multidimensional nature of need, encompassing aspects of the quality of life, the absence or presence of well-being, the role of socio-economic and structural factors, and subjectively defined need.[8–10] This view of need has been less prominent within the NHS but has gained increasing recognition alongside policy drives such as the 'Local Voices' initiative.

The lack of a coherent approach to needs definition within the NHS has evoked some criticism. Seedhouse, for example, has commented that needs assessment activities 'tend to be disparate, varying in accordance with local factors and interests – an inevitable consequence of the lack of a reasoned, practically specific definition of need' (p. 28).[5] In an editorial on need, Culyer also notes that if the concept of 'need' is to be of practical utility then the value content of the term needs to 'be upfront and easily interpretable'.[11]

Within primary care, the lack of clarity about need definition within the NHS more generally is accentuated. Recent policy documents on primary care have emphasized a 'clinical perspective' on need, whilst at the same time stressing the requirement for primary care to be able to respond to 'vague' and 'undifferentiated problems' and to be responsive to patients' needs. 'Inappropriate demand', particularly with regard to 'out-of-hours' services, has also been a focus of discussion about need and demand within primary care.

INAPPROPRIATE DEMAND FOR PRIMARY CARE SERVICES

Concern about 'inappropriate demand' has been fuelled by evidence of increasing demand for out-of-hours services. How much such increases are a result of patient demand, or changes in remuneration and practices on the part of primary care professionals, is a moot point.[12] Nonetheless, the use of such services has understandably concentrated attention on how to manage and reduce patient demand.

Operationalizing 'inappropriateness' for research and policy purposes is problematic. The nature of illness is such that symptoms remain uncertain for diagnosing physicians, as well as for lay people.[13] Thus, attributions of appropriateness can only be made with the wisdom of hindsight. What comes to be seen as 'inappropriate' demand is also influenced by organizational arrangements operating within the NHS. Boundary maintenance by different parts of the health system, particularly A&E services, defines to an extent who is an appropriate or inappropriate user within the primary care sector.[14]

The literature relevant to 'inappropriate demand' in primary care extends to types of consulting patient, consequences for the practitioner of dealing with inappropriate consulters and imputed causes and solutions to the problem. Key findings from the literature are that:

* studies of general practice carried out in the 1960s and 1970s conceptualized the problem of inappropriateness as the presentation of 'trivial' problems whilst more recent analyses have added to this formulation by incorporating the phenomenon of the 'heartsink' or 'difficult' patient[15-18]
* consultations by certain kinds of patient are considered more appropriate than others. 'Appropriate' consulters include: those who are anxious, elderly or very young; those with mobility problems or those who would suffer severe distress from not

visiting the doctor; and patients who repeatedly consult with persistent illness. 'Inappropriate' consulters refer to those who are culturally or socially very different from the doctor; and those whose consultations stem from family rather than individual problems[17,19,20]

- both past and recent studies estimate 'inappropriate' consultations to constitute about a quarter of all attendances by patients
- considerations of appropriate demand, according to standard medical criteria, in general practice are in some respects different to hospital specialists on the one hand and lay people on the other. Primary care notions of inappropriateness are therefore likely to be midway between those of lay people and specialists[21]
- primary care professionals tend to view inappropriate demand and need in a context of their own concerns about growing workloads and expectations from patients.

Existing studies of inappropriate use within primary care tend to be normative, that is, biased in favour of the subjective feelings evoked in general practitioners (GPs) by patients. For example, in one study the use of the concept of 'heartsink patient' is justified on the grounds that:

> ... while it lacks the charm of many neologisms, it is nonetheless descriptive. Ellis's term 'dysphoria' is more elegant but sanitizes a messy feeling and focuses attention away from the sufferer onto the patient. 'Heartsink' more clearly refers to the doctor's emotions which are triggered by certain patients.[18]

There is less literature on lay perspectives or from professional groups other than GPs working in primary care about what constitutes inappropriate demand or consultation. The evidence there is suggests that patients have a strong desire not to be perceived to be consulting unnecessarily. There is also some evidence that notions of appropriateness are *negotiated* during the process of doctor–patient interaction, rather than being fixed and predetermined[22–24] and that past use and experience of contact with primary care professionals are relevant to the way in which people formulate subsequent demand for services.[25] This is examined in greater detail in Chapter 6.

3

Perspectives in the study of service utilization

The normative bias of studies, which focuses on the work pressures of GPs, provides a restricted understanding of the processes which shape the relationship between health need, demand and health services use. Additionally, a problem with the social science and medical literature on need is that it rarely refers to patient decision-making and the way in which people use services. Research which addresses help-seeking specifically is of more help in this regard.

A substantial amount of literature has been developed to understand factors relevant to health care use. This includes work which has examined the relationship between symptoms (as indicators of need) and consultation rates. Another body of work, predominantly undertaken in the United States (US), has incorporated a wide range of social, psychological and economic factors in examining the relationship between need, demand and use of services. A third focus is provided by research which has understood help-seeking as a social process.

Symptoms as an explanation
for help-seeking

Unreported symptoms have been conceptualized in epidemiological literature as 'a clinical iceberg'. The iceberg metaphor relates to reported (above water) and unreported (below water) symptoms. These clinical iceberg studies represent a traditional symptom-based means of identifying the gap between health need and demand for services. A number of studies have sought to estimate the proportion of symptoms that result in consultation with primary care and/or to explore the type of symptoms involved in consultation compared to non-consultation. Studies over a number of years have found that only a small proportion of health problems experienced by individuals are seen by medical practitioners in primary care. This literature suggests that the ratio of unreported to consulted symptoms varies according to the type of symptom experienced. For example, there is less under-reporting for severe symptoms than more minor ones.[26-30]

The focus on symptoms as the main explanatory factor in consulting behaviour has a number of limitations. There is competing evidence which suggests that neither the type nor the severity of symptoms are in themselves adequate explanations for individual decision-making in relation to help-seeking. For example, there are disagreements both amongst professional and between professional and lay people over the notions of the existence and interpretation of biophysical reality. Mechanic has argued that symptom-reporting reflects a pattern of illness behaviour which is influenced largely by the affective state of the individual.[31] Existing methodologies are also inadequate for clarifying whether differences lie in bodily sensations or in the socially constructed meaning attached to these by patients.

There is some evidence within the literature for counter-intuitive patterns of service use in relation to long-standing or chronic conditions. Studies suggest that formal health care use for chronic conditions is subject to fluctuation and may even decrease over time. For example, Bendelow's qualitative study[32] of the careers of patients with chronic pain showed that a significant number of patients accommodated to their symptoms by the self-management of pain. Patient strategies, reinforced by lower expectations of services through service contact over time, played a more important role in the management of symptoms than accessing and using formal health care services.[30] The limitations of the symptom-based model are addressed by other approaches to explaining the use of services.

TRADITIONAL MODELS OF HEALTH CARE USE

Over the last three decades, the health belief model (HBM), the rational choice model (RCM) and socio-behavioural model have been the dominant theories of utilization. These models and related studies were mainly developed in the US where access to services has been more of a salient research and policy issue than in the United Kingdom (UK). These models have also been developed and used in relation to a variety of other, different, health care systems.[33–35]

Health belief model

Individual decisions made by patients entering care are the focus of the HBM from within health psychology (and the RCM from within health economics – see below). Studies which have drawn upon the HBM have focused on exploring the characteristics of groups using health services. This model has been developed to take account of four sets of variables attributable to individual help-seeking, which are then correlated with whether or not help is sought. The four sets of variables are:

(1)   readiness to take a particular course of action
(2)   perceived risks and benefits from uptake of health care

(3) internal and external cue to action (e.g. internal cues like pain or external ones such as interference with everyday life)
(4) modifying factors (e.g. gender, age, ethnicity, class, personality).

In general terms, research using this model suggests that high users of services perceive themselves to be ill and vulnerable to illness while low users of primary care express less anxiety about illness and are less concerned about symptoms. Perceived severity of illness and susceptibility to illness have been viewed as a relevant factor in the initiation of the use of primary care. Low users of primary care are more likely to be critical and less convinced of the efficacy and benefits of medical treatments. Similarly, the association of traits with low use are at times associated with those patients GPs find 'difficult' to deal with, and high users fit more into the ideal type of 'compliant patients'. Perceived susceptibility has been found to be a predictor of attendance for health check-ups.[36,37] Those who are high users of primary care prevention services and those who are more likely to use medically dependent health promotion screening also appear more likely to adopt a 'doctor knows best' attitude and to perceive themselves as having lower personal control over their health. An interesting research question is whether perceived susceptibility to illness increases or decreases more generally in primary care amongst those identified as having personality traits which are associated with being high users of primary care prevention services.

A closely related set of studies within the HBM tradition use the concepts of 'locus of control' and 'coping', which are also important for understanding help-seeking and self-management and care. However, there is a dearth of studies which relate these concepts to illness behaviour and the use of primary or secondary care services. Most concentrate on preventative health promotion or screening services.

The rational choice model

The RCM of decision-making is prominent in the health economics literature and has been adopted in research seeking to understand health care decisions more generally. It also forms a central focus of the HBM just discussed. From this perspective, lay decisions are viewed as 'purposive' and as being made by individual social actors who weigh up the costs and benefits of a particular action in situations with variable characteristics, constraints and opportunities.[38] The model assumes that, in making a decision, people begin by determining whether they stand to win or lose according to some reference point. The RCM has been used most extensively in examining decisions made by patients or lay people in a health care context but in areas which are relatively distant to primary care, such as specialist interventions.

Socio-behavioural utilization model

Within the social medicine literature, a 'pathways' model has gained considerable popularity as a way of shedding light on patterns of motivation for use of services. In relation to medical consultation for minor physical and psychological problems, a number of researchers have used path analysis within a behavioural model in an attempt to understand differential levels of access among subgroups of the US and other European country populations.[39–41] The basis of this type of model rests on three sets of factors (Figure 3.1) which constitute the foundation of individual, rational decision-making:

(1) *predisposing factors* – the predisposition to use services suggested by demographic, social characteristics and beliefs about services
(2) *enabling factors* – the concern here is with issues of access to care and the organizational characteristics of the health

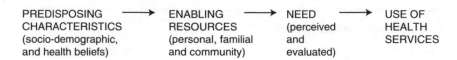

Figure 3.1: Socio-behavioural model.[41]

system. Enabling characteristics reflect the available means, knowledge and ability to act, needed to use health care. These include: geographical availability, having a consistent and regular source of care, travel time and financial ability, which limits or promotes the use of services

(3) *need factors* – these relate to the nature of the illness and include type and severity of symptoms. They refer to both biophysical aspects and social and psychological aspects such as the hurt, worry and bother a condition may cause.

LIMITATIONS OF TRADITIONAL UTILIZATION MODELS

It is obviously easier to study or to treat the individual and even easier to blame the individual for health problems or failures to seek medical care promptly, than to consider problems of health in a more inclusive framework.[42]

Traditional models of health care use provide a set of extensive contingencies ranging from the psychological – for example, patient preferences in the health belief model – to the external environment, including the policy context, in the social-behavioural model. However, these types of models of health use have certain limitations. They can be subjected to critical scrutiny on the basis that:

• there is an inbuilt assumption to view all utilization action as choice and to ignore the importance of habitual behaviour

- there is a failure to account for the potential impact of social networks on seeking care from formal services
- they concentrate on the outcome of the decision rather than the decision-making process
- they are best for accounting for acute conditions requiring hospitalization and therefore are less relevant for accounting for chronic-illness trajectories, use of care over time and primary health and social care which is community orientated
- the importance of social variables is rarely explored in detail. The social characteristics of those using services are restricted to describing the cross-sectional relationship between social position and consultation rates. The identification of the socio-demographic characteristics of a group tells us little about why those in a particular grouping may be more or less likely to consult services
- because of the concentration on statistical associations they cannot adequately take into account the purposeful actions and meanings of individuals in seeking help and making decisions.

4

Help-seeking and
health care as a
social process

*Service use (is) not a single, yes–no, one-time decision but patterns
and pathways of practices and people consulted during an illness
episode. Patterns of care describe the combination of advisors and/or
practices that are used during the course of an illness episode. Pathways add the additional element of order, that is, the sequences of
advisors and/or practices used over the course of an illness episode.*

*[Pescosolido and Boyer (1996) describing the network–episode
model.]*[43]

SOCIAL PROCESS MODELS

Research on the process of decision-making from within medical
sociology and social psychology has tended to move away from
motivation and determinants of decision-making as fixed attri-
butes of the individual. Instead, this work focuses on the *interaction*
of the patient with others and views the motivation and determin-
ance of decision-making as subject to the influence of a wide range

of factors which are often beyond an individual's control. A number of approaches can be incorporated within this tradition. An early departure from traditional health utilization studies is the *illness career approach* which developed within medical sociology and anthropology as an alternative to the correlational models. Understanding the ways in which the patient role is negotiated and maintained and how others react to and categorize illness, concepts of self and identity, stages of a medical consultation, psychological and personal change and phases of hospitalization characterize this approach. Of most relevance to widening our understanding of help-seeking is the centrality of the experience of illness. The latter is viewed as being embedded in a set of logical, critical decision points which are nonetheless flexible and where 'alternative decisions at any step can lead to further decision or to a reconsideration of earlier ones'.[44] Pescosolido has recently added to these previous conceptualizations of 'illness as a career model' by viewing lay health decision-making as rooted in a process whereby decisions made at any stage are shaped by those made at an earlier stage.

During the 1960s and 1970s a number of models of lay referral were developed as a means of understanding help-seeking behaviour. These elaborated on the stages or pathways into care. An early example of the process of referral is provided by a study conducted by Zola and colleagues in which five non-physiological triggers to the referral process were identified:[45]

(1) the occurrence of an interpersonal crisis
(2) perceived interference with personal and/or social relationships
(3) the 'sanctioning' of ill health by others
(4) perceived interference with work-related activities
(5) temporalizing of symptoms, e.g. 'If it doesn't get better by ... I'll see a doctor'.

Since that time further work has been undertaken which illuminates the relevance of a range of factors and processes on health service use. The amount of empirical work in this area is not great, but what there is suggests the importance of the process of decision-making rather than the decision itself, the conceptualization of illness as inherently social in nature, the involvement of others in decision-making and the social context of decision-making. In this regard, motivation and other determinants of decision-making are frequently seen as lying beyond an individual's control. Studies of help-seeking have identified the relevance of examining:

- the timing between onset of problems and consultation
- the extent to which people are able to contain and cope with signs and symptoms within socially defined situations and contexts. For example, Alonzo's studies of people's illness management suggest that where individuals are able to contain signs and symptoms within their everyday situations, these will not reach medical attention.[42,46] The ability of people to contain symptoms within a range of social situations is considered to be influenced by a number of contextualized factors, including the commitment to and engrossment in these situations, tolerance of illness behaviour by others, power relationships among participants and coping resources
- the multiple possibilities in the decision-making process, including the overturning of decisions, and non-decision-making as well as the reasons for seeking out formal help
- the relationship between everyday events, activities, work and decisions to use primary care.

There is a complex and paradoxical relationship between work, service use and illness behaviour. The perceived interference of symptoms with work performance can operate as a trigger to medical consultation. At other times, work may act to prevent the seeking of help. In high-risk occupational settings the range of signs and symptoms that need to be contained is high but so is the threshold of containment. Engrossment in and commitment to work predispose people to contain the symptoms of illness, thus delaying or even preventing help-seeking from formal services.[42] In a study of illness behaviour amongst residents of a lodging house, Bloor found that people sought to guard their work routines against disruptions by illness and that 'the exigencies of the work situation led workers to seek to accommodate illness at least on a short-term basis' (p. 307).[47] Similarly, Cowie found that a number of people he had interviewed who had experienced myocardial infarctions attempted to complete routine tasks in which they were engaged when their heart attacks were happening.[48] Finally, the importance of work as a factor in people's help-seeking is reflected in studies which show the value that some groups place on the provision of practical and tangible support that GPs are able to provide in easing employment situations.[49]

BRIDGING THE GAP BETWEEN MODELS OF USE

An emerging generation of health-utilization studies and models, e.g. the network–episode model (NEM) and the social organization strategy model, promises to bridge a gap between individualistic and social-process models of decision-making.[38,43,50] Social interaction and social networks are incorporated into the mechanisms for seeking help, together with notions of purposive action, economic and psychological rationality and 'utility maximization', drawn from the rational choice model of decision-making. (The latter – utility maximization – is viewed as a mechanism through which people learn about, comprehend and try to deal with difficulties.) This approach is predicated on the assumption of heterogeneity amongst groups of individuals who seek help from medical practitioners and the power of social networks to influence service use. The focus of this approach is not only on who accesses care but *when* and *how* care is received and a central question raised by this model is how are choices and strategies relating to help-seeking socially organized? The potential of the NEM, which also encapsulates the main advantages of using a social process model more generally and is particularly suited to understanding use in community contexts, has been described by Pescosolido and Boyer as follows:

> *The NEM contends that patterns and pathways are embedded in social life, in the context of personal lives and changing communities. Illness careers do not occur in a vacuum. People's ongoing social lives are depicted in the social support system. Individuals are seen as both pragmatic and faced with social contingencies. Rejecting the idea of rational choice does not mean the individuals have to be seen as irrational puppets of their environment. Rather, they have a great deal of common-sense knowledge and cultural routines held from past experience, from talking to others, and from others offering advice when unusual behaviour occurred. These encounters can be short or momentary, planned or spontaneous, supportive or controversial.*[43]

Though there is a substantial body of empirical work in progress in the area of mental health, to date the writings about the possibilities of NEM are more substantial than the empirical findings generated by the use of the models. The relevance of the NEM model for understanding primary care is that it situates an understanding of the management of illness in a context which incorporates elements of formal/informal health care resources and which works across the interfaces between service sectors (Figure 4.1).

In addition to the models described above, a number of themes can be identified from the literature which have implicit relevance to the formulation of need, demand and use of care. These are discussed further in Chapter 5.

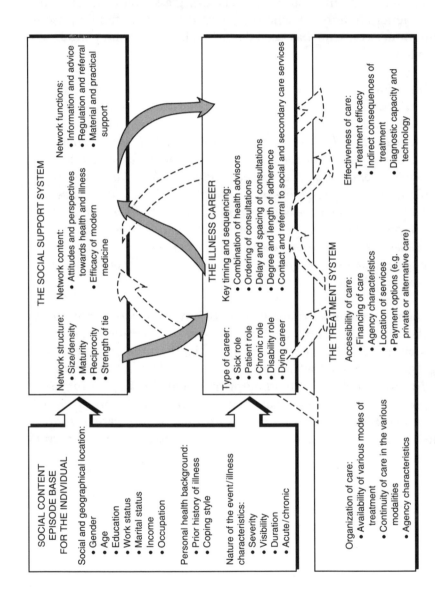

Figure 4.1: Network–episode model (adapted).[50]

5

The relevance of
lay concepts and
experience of illness
for help-seeking

There is a dialectical relationship between use of services and lay
views of health and illness. People's notions of health and illness
and past experience of the use of services seem to have an influence on the process of decision-making and help-seeking. In turn,
the impact of directly using services shapes views about treatment,
professionals and illnesses. Qualitative research on lay peoples'
conceptions of illness and the contextual bases of their response to
the experience of illness has also extended to examining how individuals ascertain that they are ill. The place of feeling in illness
and its potential importance in the social organization of lay
and professional primary care has been illustrated by the work of
Telles and Pollack.[51] In past studies of health beliefs, there has been
a tendency to overdraw the difference between lay and medical conceptions of health and illness. More recent analyses have pointed
to overlaps in, and shared use of, terms and societal values between
professionals and lay groups. However, one difference between
clinical and lay perspectives suggested by qualitative research is
the different interpretations and meanings attributed to the use of
similar medical terms.[52] For example, in relation to the presentation
of chronic illness such as musculoskeletal disorders in primary care,

lay people have been found to utilize a rich indepth vocabulary to describe the experience of symptoms which extends beyond the medical description and diagnosis of lower back pain (see Borkan *et al.*).[53] The use of qualitative research such as this needs to be extended to other groups in the population where views and actions within a primary care context have received less attention.

LAY CONCEPTS OF ILLNESS, ILLNESS BEHAVIOUR AND HELP-SEEKING

Three themes relevant to the issue of help-seeking and service use were identified from the literature on lay conceptions of health and illness.

1. *The lay evaluation of symptoms and risk factors.* The lay assessment of symptoms and risk is important in understanding the timing and nature of the use of primary care services.

Helen Roberts' ethnographic study of parents' use of accident and emergency services illustrates the relationship between risk assessment and the use of services. She found that parents' accounts of the assessment of illness management centred on 'being on the safe side' in the context of not being able to predict the outcome of an illness episode and beliefs about the responsibilities of 'being a good mother'. Parents used A&E services in relation to assessments of what might happen rather than on the evaluation of existing behaviour or sign and symptoms of illness.[54]

2. *Concepts of health and illness as imperatives or inhibitors of help-seeking.* A number of studies have identified a moral imperative ingrained in both lay and medical constructs of health and illness which places a high value on stoicism and 'not complaining'. The assumption is that these values are likely to inhibit referral and are conducive to the toleration of, rather than help-seeking for, symptoms. However, the relationship of these values to patient-consulting practices has rarely been examined empirically. One older and one

recent study illustrate the links that can be made between lay conceptions of illness and use of primary care services.

Firstly, Williams made a link between the nature of cross-cultural lay logic and the use of primary care services. The configuration of service provision is seen as impacting on lay notions of illness as a dialectical process. Williams noted the cultural differences in the weight attributed to strength and weaknesses in the realm of health and illness by Scottish and French people. For Scottish respondents, functional fitness was viewed as dependent on the freedom from a disabling disease and not on strength. In contrast, strength was central to French respondents' notions of health. In light of the observation that French GPs handled twice the rate of psychosomatic complaints as their British counterparts and were more lavish in their prescribing habits – particularly of tonics and vitamins – Williams suggested that the practice of medical consultation in the two countries may be related to lay conceptions.[55]

Secondly, Salmon and his colleagues examined health beliefs in relation to the presentation of common primary care ailments. Beliefs about symptoms of patients attending their GPs were compared across three types (respiratory, musculoskeletal and gastrointestinal). Developing insights from qualitative sociology and anthropology using Q methodology, eight belief dimensions were formulated into scales: stress, lifestyle, 'wearing out', environment, internal–structural, internal–functional, weak constitution, concern. Gastrointestinal symptoms were the most likely to be attributed to internal malfunctions and lifestyle or weak constitution. Musculoskeletal symptoms were more likely to be attributed to structural problems caused by the body 'wearing out' and respiratory symptoms to the influence of the environment. This formulation by Salmon and his colleagues is likely to be of significant utility in examining the relationship between beliefs and patterns of use of services over time.[56]

3. *The ways in which understanding of health and illness is linked to people's environment in ways which have an indirect impact on decision-making and help-seeking.* Past studies of lay conceptions of

illness have focused almost exclusively on analysing the narratives and accounts of patients. Recent studies of patient–doctor communication have shown that constructs of health and illness are, in part, an outcome of interaction between health professionals and patients. For example, in a recent study of medical encounters a characteristic narrative structure and sequencing of the consultation had the effect of marginalizing the contextual aspects of patients' problems and reinforcing ideas of stoicism and individualism.[57] It seems essential therefore that the consultation becomes a key focus for research which seeks to understand the relationship between lay conceptions of illness, health need and patterns of care.

THE PAST USE OF SERVICES AND ITS IMPACT ON SUBSEQUENT UTILIZATION

A small number of studies point to the relevance of past experience of services and professionals as influences on subsequent decisions to use services. There is some evidence that help-seeking is shaped by an assessment of what can and cannot be done, based on prior contact with services. While most studies of satisfaction with services do not make a link between satisfaction with care and subsequent use, the connections between beliefs, attitudes, knowledge, expectations, experience of, and satisfaction with, services and help-seeking behaviour are likely to be intricate. This is illustrated by two studies.

Firstly, in a study of the last year of life of 785 people who died in the UK in 1969, the researchers found that many of the individuals had not sought medical assistance for their symptoms. Comments made by relatives suggested that the explanation for people's failure to consult lay in their realistic assessment of the degree to which doctors could help.[58]

Secondly, in a qualitative study of the management of cystitis in primary care, Pill argued that the nature of the experience of the consultation feeds back into how women perceive and manage subsequent episodes of symptoms. Contact with the doctor enabled women to put a label on their symptoms, but doctors' frequent use of the infection model and their emphasis on the random nature of the attacks tended to limit the control women felt they could exercise in managing the condition. This appeared to be compounded by a reported lack of information about the diagnosis that was being made. There was little attempt to elicit women's own ideas about what was wrong and little reinforcement of self-help measures. Thus the experience of seeing a doctor for an ailment at one point in time may increase the likelihood of future help-seeking.[25]

6

The relevance of
social networks to
help-seeking

Many individuals (also) consult friends, relatives and others in a
lay referral system where a doctor is only one of many specialists.[59]

Research which has examined the impact of social networks on
help-seeking is small compared to the extensive social research
which explores the relationship between social ties and morbidity.
What research exists tends to be inconclusive. Reviewed overall,
research findings are inconsistent and differ according to condition, type of health action, population group and context under
investigation.[60] While some social scientists have been enthusiastic
proponents of the importance of the lay referral system, there are
also indications from the literature that the presence or absence of
social networks are not good predictors of utilization, or are only
of significance in combination with other factors. Recent analysis
has pointed to the need to extend the metaphor of networks to
formal health care providers in a bid to understand how professional ties coalesce with lay networks in the use of services.[50]

Qualities of social networks such as size, interconnectedness,
activity, maturity, proximity, membership and supportiveness
have all been found to be associated with health care use. These

qualities vary across population groups. Of most significance are differences between men and women. Women dominate lay networks both as health users and resource providers and are more likely to facilitate access to professional care and exercise greater control over network members' health behaviours than men.[61]

The literature suggests that social networks influence help-seeking in a number of ways by:

- acting as a buffer to the experience of stress, which reduces or eliminates the need for help
- acting as screening and referral agents to professional services
- transmitting attitudes, values and norms about help-seeking
- precluding the need for professional support by providing instrumental and affective support.

The role of social networks in referral varies depending on the relationship between the individuals involved.[62] The nature of the impact on decision-making is also diverse. To an extent, lay networks operate by providing confirmative action and advice as an adjunct to individual decision-making. The nature of the relationship between the person seeking advice and the lay referrer and the provision of social support provides some insight into the reasons for diversity in the way social networks operate as screening and referral agents. Older people are more likely to rely on carers to make referral decisions than other groups.[63] Members of individuals' social network who are not family members are less likely to tolerate delays in help-seeking due to normalization or denial of symptoms. Neighbours and friends may have a lower threshold for contacting services because of the moral responsibility of taking risks with other people's health. In some instances it has been found that help-seeking from formal services may be motivated by the presence rather than absence of social networks.[64–67]

There are also groups of people who can be viewed as midway between lay referral networks and professional services. These include the clergy, police officers and non-health-attached social workers. The main way in which these groups operate is as a filtering system to formal services. However, despite the likely significance of these 'public process personnel', empirical evidence for their influence in the screening and processing of referrals to primary care is notable by its absence.[64]

7

Individual self-care

and lay care provided

by others

... one of the most frequently encountered, unresolved disputes concerns the potential consequences of increased lay responsibility for health-related matters. One point on which there is agreement, however, is the fact that our present knowledge of self-care is fragmentary and a great deal of further investigation is required.[68]

An important, but often hidden, aspect of the demand and supply of health care is the provision of individual self-care provided by others. Existing research on self-care may also underestimate its prevalence because of the way sickness absence from employment has been conceptualized as a *need*, instead of a demand reduction strategy.[64] There is some evidence which suggests that staying off work is an effective form of health care. Most of the survey studies on self-care and lay management of illness appear to have emerged over the last two decades and have been undertaken in Canada, the United States and Northern Europe.[68–72] Additionally, these studies and others illustrate the considerable range of non-medication activities used by lay people in response to illness.[73–75] A number of commentators have stressed the empowering and positive aspects of lay management in allowing individuals to take more control over their own lives and health.[72] There is also evidence that lay management of care can reduce reliance on health professionals. However, the positive gains and assumed potential of self-care to reduce health expenditure has, according to some, been exaggerated. Some have pointed to its excessive individualism and there is concern over the 'victim-blaming potential' of the emphasis on self-help and the lack of resources of those in most need to provide and reciprocate informal care for themselves and others.

Individual self-care arises as an option out of many when experiencing symptoms. Suggestions from the literature are that people do what is pragmatic and generally choose multiple treatments, conventional and alternative, in dealing with episodes of illness. These illness behaviours include:

- decisions to do nothing about symptoms
- self-medication
- non-medication self-treatment
- decisions to consult professional providers (as discussed above).

Choices are, in turn, shaped by socio-demographic influences and the situations that people find themselves in.

Non-health action

In comparison to the other three areas of illness behaviour, relatively little is known about the extent to which people decide to do nothing about identified illness, although there is some evidence that this varies according to the type of symptoms experienced. Estimates from surveys conducted in other countries suggest that one-third of conditions have not been treated in any way and that non-action is a relevant strategy when dealing with both acute/ temporary and longer-term conditions.[69] There is some evidence to suggest that no-action responses to symptoms may vary with age as well as condition. Non-action in relation to asthma, for example, has been associated with teenagers more than other groups in the population.

Non-action in relation to the presence of symptoms has been interpreted in a variety of ways. The failure to obtain treatment for untreated symptoms has been attributed to negative psychological traits on the part of individuals and a means of personal control and coping people adopt. An American study by Thompson et al.[76] suggests that in relation to some illnesses, such as cancer, it is important for patients to believe that they can control daily emotional reactions and physical symptoms. From a lay perspective, there is some evidence that the presence of symptoms is regarded as a normal part of everyday life. Stoicism and self-reliance are also relevant constructs to non-action insofar as they are related to the need for privacy and the threat of disclosure.[55]

SELF-MEDICATION

Self-medication has received the most attention in the literature on self-care.[70,77] Self-medication with non-prescribed medication has been found to exceed the use of prescription drugs and refers to:

- the use of substances considered to maintain health or prevent illness
- the treatment of self-limiting conditions or early stages of more serious illness
- treatment taken in addition to professionally prescribed medication.

Homeopathic and herbal remedies have increased significantly in recent years and are frequently taken in the absence of consultation with an alternative therapist. The psychosocial characteristics of self-reliance have been associated with self-medication.[70] In terms of the reasons lay people give for self-medication practices, one study suggests that control over the therapeutic process and self-knowledge is likely to be a more important variable at times than perceived efficacy. People appear to use self- and formal medication in response to situations which arise as part of everyday life. For example, there is some evidence that the retention of prescribed drugs for future use is a common practice.[71] A sense of autonomy, self-control and choice is central to this type of use and, because of this, a more sceptical attitude to the taking of drugs is also associated with this pattern of use. In the research literature, the use of home remedies (e.g. drinks, rubs, herbs) is sometimes seen as a continuum of self-medication practices. However, at other times they receive separate consideration.

Non-medication self-treatment

Non-medication self-treatment incorporates a wide range of practices. The four identified studies which were directly concerned with exploring the use of home remedies found a far higher rate of use than those studies that did not have such a specific focus but included them as a general category.[68,71,78,79] Additionally, these studies and others illustrate the considerable range of non-medication activities used by lay people in response to illness. Items which have been identified in the literature include: alteration of diet; the taking of, or changing of, exercise regimen; rest/bed rest; having a holiday; reducing workload; taking fresh air; poultices; and the use of appliances such as heat pads. Also included under the rubric of non-medication action are aspects of self-care which can be categorized as 'coping behaviour' in the general management of stress. Habits of stress reduction coupled with beliefs regarding the factors which determine health have been found to influence both the ways in which symptoms are perceived and patterns of illness behaviour.

Estimates of the level of use of home remedies are difficult to find and those that do exist differ widely in accordance with the definition and value attributed to home remedies as a form of health action. Some definitions limit self-treatment to home appliances, herbal medications and various forms of home remedies. This narrow conceptualization has been criticized for approximating self-care to the medical model and potentially excluding some beneficial forms of self-care.[71] Other researchers have extended the notion to other aspects of everyday life, such as seeing family or friends, or going out for lunch.[78] Using the latter definition of self-care behaviour requires taking into consideration the presence of other people.

SOCIO-DEMOGRAPHIC AND SITUATIONAL INFLUENCES

Research suggests that situational constraints and socio-demographic variations have an influence on the use of home remedies and non-medication self-care. Those with low household incomes, fewer years of education and lower social-class groups more frequently maintained their normal routines when ill with influenza, while respondents in higher social-class groups more frequently remained at home or undertook bed rest.[68,80] The use of remedies also appears to be generationally and culturally linked, with older generations preferring to use traditional home remedies and younger generations turning to propriety medicines. While 'traditional' home remedies have declined there is some evidence to suggest that homeopathic and herbal medicines are used more extensively among younger and middle-aged groups.[81]

THE LAY–PROFESSIONAL INTERFACE IN SELF-MANAGEMENT

Interest has recently been shown, from health care professionals, in the potential of self-care practices – particularly for conditions such as asthma and diabetes – which raises a number of interesting issues about how the interface between self- and professionally-provided care is configured and managed. While some have welcomed this interest as a means of promoting efficient and autonomous health care, some commentators have pointed to the threat of professional co-option and medicalization of self-care practices. This assertion is supported to some extent by analysis of self-care material which reflects dominant medical values and norms. Nonetheless, probably the most relevant question to ask about self-care with regard to the contemporary primary care agenda is 'What is the potential for combining the skills and practices of lay and professional primary care providers?'. At present, there is a dearth of research with which to begin to answer this question. However, one recently completed NPCRDC study which begins to explore this issue has shown that for the treatment of minor ailments, the public use the community pharmacy as an alternative to the GP, and that the advice-giving role of pharmacist staff, to an extent, reinforces and promotes self-care practices.[82]

LAY CARE PROVIDED BY OTHERS

What we do not have is a well-based understanding of how carers fit into the service system, and how their needs are, and are not, incorporated into the practice of mainstream service providers.[83]

The notion of care provided by lay others, and its relationship to formal primary care services, is a complex one. It is not clear whether such care acts as a supplement or alternative to formal service provision, although in other areas of research there is evidence that it operates in both of these ways. In relation to the use of services by elderly people, research based on a compensatory model provides evidence that formal services are used only as a last resort when informal resources are unavailable, and other research suggests that lay advice and care promotes the use of services.[84]

While a vast literature exists on lay or informal care, little was identified which was linked directly to the issues of health need and demand for primary-care services. One of the rare studies which has made a direct connection between care provided by others and access to, and use of, primary care is research undertaken in the context of an investigation of access to employment opportunities and health services in deprived areas of Merseyside. Findings suggested that complex arrangements and negotiations are required before health decisions can be acted upon, of which substitute care arrangements for dependants is one consideration. Respondents were found to request help from other households to look after vulnerable dependants whilst contact was made with primary care services. Relatively scarce resources, available from other households, were saved up for crises or appointments seen as more serious. This may affect the use of primary health-care visits which are perceived as more routine and involve less travel and waiting time. Inter-household favours were often sought reluctantly, respondents 'rationing' the circumstances in which they would call on substitute care, and the borrowing of time was used in relation to those perceived to be in most need. Within this scheme, women's own health needs were often given a low priority.[67]

The literature on social support and care provided by self-help groups has indirect relevance to help-seeking in primary care.

SOCIAL SUPPORT

Social support refers to emotional, instrumental and affirmational support as well as advocacy assistance. These have been related in turn to different combinations of network provision. Social support has been found to promote indirectly the self-coping behaviour of vulnerable individuals – much of this work is undertaken from a psychological perspective – with some studies reporting a relationship between positive means of coping and social support.[85] Aspects which have most relevance for a greater understanding of patterns of use of formal primary services are:

- people's perceptions of social support, including the *perceived* availability as well as the direct effects of social support, which have been found to have a direct positive effect on future coping
- the role of social support as a supplement or alternative to professional care. While a number of studies have examined the impact of social support on self-coping, there has been less emphasis on the process and mediating effects of social support in relation to the formulation of need and demand for services.[86]

SELF-HELP GROUPS

The benefits of self-help groups which have proliferated in the health care arena in recent years include the provision of mutual aid, information and support. These groups have been viewed as providing sources of supplementary support outside patients' existing social networks and a means of sharing long-term existential problems through emphatic mutual support. The proliferation of self-help groups at a time of expansion in formal health care provision suggests that they address problems which are either neglected or inadequately dealt with by professional services. In the literature, the campaigning role of such groups in attempting to influence the health care system has also been viewed as a form of self-care. In Norway, many patient organizations provide information about the quality of the practitioners. The rise of these groups points to extensive patient responsibility for health in the context of:

- the failure of existing services to meet self-defined need
- increasing recognition of the value of mutual help alongside or as an alternative to professional help

• highlighting self-help and alternative responses to the management of illness.

At a cultural level, too, it is likely that the formation of self-help and campaigning groups has had an impact on demand for services. This is particularly the case for new or disputed illness categories which are encountered first within the formal health services sector by primary care. Some groups, such as those concerned with chronic fatigue syndrome (ME), have been drivers for demands on services and policy-makers to respond to emergent needs.[86-91]

8

Organizational factors influencing demand for, and use of, services

The new agenda must link individuals in all their social-psychological complexity to institutions and social context in all their structural complexity.[92]

In addition to population factors and attendant social processes, supply or organizational factors are of relevance to the demand and use of services. In his 1972 review of health care utilization, McKinlay points to a preoccupation in health care utilization studies with identifying and labelling individual characteristics in population groups as the main way of understanding the use or non-use of services.[3] In contrast, organizational phenomena which are also related to utilization behaviour were considered to be an omission within the literature. For McKinlay, the actions of professionals and organizational imperatives were considered to be important variables in considering health need, demand and use of services. Additionally, the way in which patients interact with organizations (client–agent/agency interaction) has been found to be influential in a number of studies. In relation to more contemporary debates about the management of demand for health care policy, discussions lean towards a concern with examining *demand* factors.[6,93]

Supply factors, whilst acknowledged as having importance in shaping, defining or legitimizing patient demand for services, are generally viewed as affecting demand and the way it is managed at the interface between primary and secondary care services (e.g. rationing by use of waiting lists). Service or provider character-istics are less frequently viewed as potential 'feedback' factors influencing patient behaviour in formulating demand for services. Service change has the capacity to alter images of health care systems and how people use them. This has been documented in relation to managed care in the US. With regard to British primary care services, the rapidly changing nature of service delivery, work force and purchasing and commissioning arrangements are im-portant variables to consider as potential influences on patients' help-seeking behaviour.

Although the implications of service formation and develop-ment are rarely assessed in terms of the specific impact on patient demand, a number of studies note more general changes in patient behaviour. As far as the existing literature is concerned, aspects which have the potential to act as a feedback influence on patient demand include:

- *changes in professional roles and perspectives.* Such changes in-clude new theories and models underpinning training, practice and involvement in aspects of care previously dealt with by the secondary care sector
- *organizational and service arrangements in primary, secondary and community care.* There is some evidence that characteristics of general practice are influential in shaping patient demand. Users of single-handed practices, for example, have been shown to consult more frequently and to more likely have contacted the practice out of normal working hours than patients of larger practices. At the level of secondary and community care, ser-vice provision which is no longer provided may generate demand at a primary care level
- *changing perspectives and policy on responses to 'need' within primary care.* Demand for services for those with psychological

problems and HIV may, in part, be a response to greater aware-
ness and responsiveness of primary care professionals to such
need
• *the introduction of computerized monitoring and record-keeping
  systems.* The provision of new types of services by GPs (such as
  health promotion screening) is an example of a service initiative
  designed to increase demand for a particular service but which
  may have a more general impact on patient demand for, and
  use of, primary care services.

9

The impact of information on lay decision-making

An important provider influence is the impact of information on patient decision-making. The provision of appropriate information is seen by policy-makers and practitioners as a means of promoting the 'responsible' use of primary care services and has also been recognized as a means of managing demand. Health maintenance organizations (HMOs) in the US have found the provision of information to prospective patients a useful demand strategy.[6] The primary care out-of-hours cooperative in Greenwich has used literature on self-care, devised and translated from Dutch, as a means of providing better information about the benefits and limitations of self-care measures.[94,95] This included detailed information about the signs, symptoms and self-treatment of common ailments. Central to this and the American strategy is the notion of self-care, which is an important element of patient responsibility in using services.

However, there is currently little research into what sources of information are most effective in changing people's illness behaviour in relation to primary care. Information sources in modern societies are numerous and complex and are of both an official and unofficial nature. Both need to be taken into account in understanding the impact of information on human behaviour. While a search of key databases revealed little literature of direct relevance to decision-making in primary care, there is literature on decision-making within other parts of the health care system which has indirect relevance to primary care.

INFORMATION AND PATIENT DECISION-MAKING

There are a number of benefits associated with providing information to patients. Information provision has been viewed by some as essential to involving patients in the making of informed decisions and being active participants in health care.[96-101] Positive outcomes, identified by a number of studies, include a reduction in emotional distress and anxiety when undergoing health procedures and a sense of control of their own illness.

Deficiencies in both the form and content of available patient information necessary to make informed and involved decisions are also a key theme in the literature.[96] An illustration of how a lack of information might relate to delays in seeking help is provided in a study by Bleeker and colleagues[65] in which people who had suffered a myocardial infarction and failed to access care quickly in an emergency were found to lack appropriate information about signs and symptoms and when to contact formal services. The evidence about deficiencies in information needs to be seen alongside findings from studies which suggest that lay people wish to be better informed in making key decisions about illness management. A recent review of the legal and ethical aspects of consumer health information suggests that there is a failure to share information about the risks and benefits of treatment and that health professionals may not provide the degree of information required by patients.[96]

Barriers to the assimilation and full use of information include the following.

Patient factors

The literature refers to memory, motivation, deficiencies in knowledge about the body, a lack of ability and confidence to make decisions and failure to act appropriately on information provided. The literature on patient factors rarely takes account of the subjective meanings, actions and context of those being researched.

Timing and context

The timing and context of the provision of information is important in terms of its effectiveness. This is illustrated by a study of the self-management of asthma, undertaken in Australia, which indicated that there are clear points at which information will be useful in decision-making and other points when it is likely to be ineffective. Two groups of patients, one recruited from within a primary care context (community pharmacy) and the other a hospitalized group, both expressed strong preferences for information concerning their condition. However, subjects preferred not to make decisions alone about the management of asthma exacerbations. As the asthma exacerbation increased, the desire to make decisions decreased. The authors concluded that 'while asthmatics have strong desires to be informed about their illness, they do not wish to be the prime decision-makers during an exacerbation'.[76]

Professional and communication factors

These include a failure to provide accurate clinical and preventative advice, a lack of communication skills among health professionals, incomprehensibility of information and a failure to address the specific needs of different population groups. Finally, information on evidence-based medicine appears to be targeted almost exclusively at health professionals, suggesting a failure to target evidence-based information to patients. In the context of wide variations in medical practice, Coulter has argued for better information about the effectiveness of medical interventions, derived from well-conducted outcome studies.[99]

The transmission of information

Another factor related to the failure of information to impact on decision-making is the effectiveness of the mode of transmission. Printed information which is adequately written is commonly accepted as the simplest and most effective means of providing information to a large number of people. However, personalized educational material has been shown to be more effective in enhancing health knowledge than non-personalized information. Studies have found that using face-to-face contact or video-taped information is more successful than using printed information. There is also some evidence to suggest the need to provide information more than once and of the positive role of new computer technology in promoting the assimilation of material by patients.[101] Finally, the importance and growing strengths of lay associations and the development of their role as information banks have been found to be effective means of ensuring standards of care and providing ongoing patient education. The means of transmitting information in this way is most developed in the US.[96]

The mass media

The public rely heavily on the mass media for information about key health issues of relevance to primary care and to influence health behaviour, health care utilization and health care practices and policy. In terms of the impact of media reports on primary care demand, one salient issue is the extent to which consultations with primary care increase after a health 'scare'. The coverage of risk is also deemed important in influencing patient response to, and construction of, health and illness problems; and the transmission and use of information have been identified as having important roles to play in promoting or inhibiting health service utilization and the formulation of patient demand. There has been no systematic exploration of the impact of coverage of primary care-relevant issues in the UK. Most analysis of the media remains fixed on secondary care services and medical technology. Nonetheless, there is a wide-ranging literature which highlights areas which need exploring in relation to primary care use and illuminates the importance of information for lay understanding and decision-making.

10

Implications for

future research

A wide-ranging literature has illustrated a myriad of factors which are implicated in shaping the relationship between health need, demand and use of services. Future research needs to develop an understanding of the interaction of these factors in the context of contemporary and anticipated developments within primary care. The following implications arise from the literature.

1. *Research on the formulation of demand and use of services should be based on the use of a social process model.* In reviewing the work on utilization it was shown that our ability to understand the actions of lay people and the processes underlying demand for, and use of, services is limited by past conceptual and methodological approaches. The focus on individual choice models has inhibited thinking which examines decision-making as a chain of events and social processes. In terms of the prerequisite for the planning of primary care services, the social process approach has the potential to map service use for illness episodes, marking temporal, spatial and thematic breaks in care. New ways of examining the way in which patients use and make decisions in contemporary primary care are required which are able to take account of the potential influence of social networks on help-seeking; the pathways to,

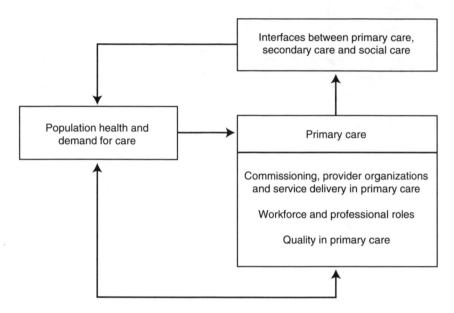

Figure 10.1: Framework for five programmes of research and development.

through and from primary care; and the relationship between people's contact with primary and secondary care professionals and the subsequent formulation of demand and use of services. A research and development strategy which addresses this wide agenda is likely to involve a multimethod, flexible and analytical approach to the study of use.

2. *Incorporating lay understandings and past experience of services with subsequent primary care use.* The relationship between concepts of health and illness and service use is a topic which requires greater exploration within primary care. The link between the experience of previous illness and service use and the management of subsequent illness episodes has relevance for understanding patterns of use in relation to 'high demand' conditions. A longitudinal design, which combined a study of patients' use of services and illness management strategies in combination with changing

professional practice, is likely to have the most relevance for primary care policy and practice.

3. *Mapping the relationship between self- and informal care and type of primary care.* Clarification is needed of the role that self- and lay management of illness plays in the formulation of demand for, and use of, formal primary care services. Does lay action substitute for, or continue alongside, formal service provision? And what types of intervention or changes in services increase or diminish the potential for self-care? Of relevance here is research which seeks to understand better the impact of different types of information on people's self-management and help-seeking activities and to consider the extent to which professional practices and skills might enhance and complement lay people's self-care.

4. *Assessing the influence of social networks and context on primary health care use.* The literature on social networks suggests that their impact on health utilization and the provision of social support is best assessed by investigating what kinds of people are involved in what networks, with references to situations at different points in the life course and different illness experience. An understanding of the interaction of lay ties with networks of primary care and other health and social care professionals is also required for the formulation of successful demand management strategies. With regard to minor ailments, the activities and roles of community pharmacists and primary care nurses are likely to be important.

5. *Research on use needs to be integrated with research on professional practice, quality and structure of primary care.* A better understanding of the factors shaping the relationship between patient demand and use of services needs to inform evaluation, research of developments and innovations in primary care provision. In particular, research which seeks to assess changes in service delivery needs to incorporate patient action and involvement in the provision of their own primary care as measurable outcomes of research-based service development. The NPCRDC's programme areas provide a rich terrain for undertaking research, which crosses the interface between formal and informal care (see Figure 10.1). The proposed

evaluation of pilot sites provides an opportunity for the realization of this research agenda.[102]

IMPLICATIONS FOR POLICY AND PRACTICE

The main purpose of this review has been to inform a research agenda-specific policy, and practice implications are dependent on the outcome of specific research projects. However, implicated in this research agenda are pointers for the development of policy. In general terms these are:

* policy approaches to need, demand and use of services require an assessment of illness as a social, as well as medical, process
* patient responsibility in the use of primary care services extends beyond encounters with health care professionals to responsibility in providing primary care to themselves and others
* there is a need to consider the scope and extent of self- and social network care provision to avoid duplication and to ensure the compatibility of health care strategies
* consideration may need to be given to the provision of some types of services (e.g. screening) within primary care which may have the paradoxical effect of increasing patient demand
* primary care purchasers and providers need to begin to address the way in which lay people might participate more fruitfully in primary care provision and decisions about health care.

As we move towards an era in primary care where commissioning and purchaser/provider arrangements require a more managed approach, understanding the nature of the formulation of demand and use of services and lay decision-making becomes central to policy-making, evaluation and health outcomes. *Primary Care: The Future* states that primary care should provide continuity of care and be properly coordinated.[103] Acceptability, responsiveness, efficiency within primary care services and the targeting of resources to achieve greater equity and balance between primary and secondary care are key aspects of the vision of a primary care-led NHS. This strategy requires an understanding of primary care services which incorporates patients' experiences of illness and use of services, and the role played in taking responsibility for their own illnesses through social networks and self-care.

Patients' perceptions are important, not only because they are a barometer of the appropriateness and effectiveness of services, but because they are a unique source of knowledge about the way in which people use services when they do for the reasons that they do. Further research which illuminates the relationship between self- and informal care, demand for, and the patterns and processes of the use of, services, has the potential to point to:

- the areas in which self-care initiatives might be promoted
- ways of enhancing the partnership between patients and professionals which promotes the most effective form of health care.

It may be that more effective working partnerships between lay people as providers of care and primary care workers circumvents referral to the secondary care sector and helps promote the more effective use of services and meeting of health need.

References

1 Ignatieff M (1984) *The Needs of Strangers*. Vintage, Berks.

2 Morris J (1967) *Uses of Epidemiology*. Churchill Livingstone, Edinburgh.

3 McKinlay J (1972) Some approaches and problems in the study of the use of services – an overview. *Journal of Health and Social Behaviour*. **13**(115): 29–46.

4 McKinlay J (1973) Social networks, lay consultation and help-seeking behaviour. *Social Forces*. **51**: 275–92.

5 Seedhouse D (1994) *Fortress NHS: A Philosophical Review of the NHS*. Wiley, Chichester.

6 Pencheon D (1996) *On Demand*. Working paper, Institute of Public Health.

7 Stevens A and Gabbay J (1991) Needs assessment. *Health Trends*. **23**: 20–3.

8 Bradshaw J (1994) The conceptualisation and measurement of need: a social policy perspective. In *Researching the People's Health* (eds J Popay and G Williams). Routledge, London.

9 Cleary P (1989) The demand and need for mental health services. In *The Future of Mental Health Services Research* (eds C Taube *et al.*) pp. 161–84.

DHS pub no (ADM) 89-1600. National Institute of Mental Health, Washington DC.

10   Doyal L and Gough I (1991) *A Theory of Human Need*. Macmillan, London.

11   Culyer A (1995) Need: the idea won't do but we still need it. *Social Science and Medicine*. **40**(6): 727–30.

12   Hallam L (1994) Primary health care outside normal working hours: review of published work. *BMJ*. **308**: 249–53.

13   Field D (1976) The social definitions of illness. In *An Introduction to Medical Sociology* (ed. D Tuckett). Tavistock, London.

14   Green J and Dale J (1992) Primary care in accident and emergency departments and general practice: a comparison. *Social Science and Medicine*. **35**(8): 987–95.

15   Cartwright A and O'Brien M (1976) Social class variations in health care and in the nature of general practice consultations. In *The Sociology of the NHS* (ed. M Stacey). Sociological Review Monograph 22. Reading 10.

16   O'Dowd T (1992) Heartsink patients optimizing care. *Practitioner*. **305**: 580.

17   Gerrard TJ and Riddell JD (1988) Difficult patients: black holes and secrets. *BMJ*. **297**: 530–2.

18   O'Dowd T (1988) Five years of heartsink patients in general practice. *BMJ*. **297**: 528–30.

19   Tuckett D, Boulton M and Olson C (1985) A new approach to the measurement of patients' understanding of what they are told in medical consultation. *Journal of Health and Social Behaviour*. **26**(1): 27–38.

20   Murray J and Williams P (1989) Self-reported illness and general practice consultations in Asian-born and British-born residents of West London. *Social Psychiatry and Psychiatric Epidemiology*. **24**(3): 143–5.

21   Horobin G (1983) Professional mystery: the maintenance of charisma. In *General Medical Practice: The Sociology of the Profession*s (eds R Dingwall and P Lewis). Routledge, London.

22   Irvine S and Cunningham-Burley S (1991) Mothers' concepts of normality, behavioural change and illness in their children. *British Journal of General Practice*. **Sept**.

23   Punamaki RL and Kokko SJ (1995) Content and predictors of consultation experiences among Finnish primary care patients. *Social Science and Medicine*. **40**(2): 231–43.

24   Rudait K (1994) *Black and Minority Ethnic Groups in England*. Health Education Authority, London.

25   Pill R (1987) Models and management: the case of cystitis in women. *Sociology of Health and Illness*. **9**(3): 265–86.

26   Vergrugge L (1985) Triggers of symptoms and health care. *Social Science and Medicine*. **20**(9): 855–76.

27   Vergrugge L and Ascione F (1987) Exploring the iceberg. Common symptoms and how people care for them. *Medical Care*. **25**: 539.

28   Stoller EP and Kart C (1995) Symptom reporting during physician consultation: results of a health diary study. *Journal of Ageing and Health*. **7**(2): 200–32.

29   Ingham J and Millar P (1982) Consulting with mild symptoms in general practice. *Social Psychiatry and Psychiatric Epidemiology*. **17**: 77-88.

30   Wadsworth M, Butterfield W and Blaney R (1971) *Health and Sickness: The Choice of Treatment*. Tavistock, London.

31   Mechanic D (1979) Correlates of physician utilization: why do major multivariate studies of physician utilization find trivial psychosocial and organizational effects? *Journal of Health and Social Behaviour*. **20**: 387.

32   Bendelow G (1996) A failure of modern medicine? Lay perspectives on a pain-relief clinic. In *Modern Medicine: Lay Perspectives and Experiences* (eds S Williams and M Calnan). UCL Press, London.

33   Kasl S and Cobb S (1966) Health behaviour, illness behaviour and sick-role behaviour. *Archives of Environmental Health*. **12**: 531–41.

34   Conrad P (1985) The meaning of medication: another look at compliance. *Social Science and Medicine*. **20**(1): 29–37.

35   Rosenstock I (1966) Why people use health services. *Milbank Memorial Fund Quarterly.* **44**: 94–106.

36   Egan K and Beaton R (1987) Response to symptoms in healthy, low utilizers of the health care system. *Journal of Psychosocial Research.* **37**: 11–21.

37   Attias J, Shemesh Z, Bleich A, Solomon Z *et al.* (1995) Psychological profile of help-seeking tinnitus patients. *Scandinavian Audiology.* **24**(1): 13–18.

38   Pescosolido B (1992) Beyond rational choice: the social dynamics of how people seek help. *American Journal of Sociology.* **97**(4): 1096–138.

39   Anderson R and Aday L (1978) Access to medical care in the US: realized and potential. *Medical Care.* **XVI**(7): 533–46.

40   Anderson J, Blue C and Lau A (1991) Women's perspective on chronic illness: ethnicity, ideology and restructuring of life. *Social Science and Medicine.* **33**(2): 101–13.

41   Anderson R (1995) Revisiting the behaviour model and accesss to care: does it matter? *Journal of Health and Social Behaviour.* **36**: 1–10.

42   Alonzo A (1984) An illness behaviour paradigm: a conceptual exploration of a situational–adaption perspective. *Social Science and Medicine.* **19**: 499–510.

43   Pescosolido B and Boyer C (1996) From the community into the treatment system – how people use health services. In *The Sociology of Mental Illness* (eds A Horwitz and T Scheid). Oxford University Press, New York.

44   Twaddle A and Hessler R (1977) *A Sociology of Health.* Misby, St Louis, Mo.

45   Zola I (1973) Pathways to the doctor: from person to patient. *Social Science and Medicine.* **7**: 77–89.

46   Alonzo A (1980) The mobile coronary care unit and the decision to seek medical care during acute episodes of coronary artery disease. *Medical Care* **18**: 297–318.

47   Bloor M (1985) Observations of abortive illness behaviour. *Urban Life.* **14**(3): 300–16.

48   Cowie W (1976) The cardiac patient's perception of his heart attack. *Social Science and Medicine*. **10**: 87–96.

49   Rogers A and Pilgrim D (1996) *Understanding and Promoting Mental Health in the Family*. Family Health Research Report, Health Education Authority.

50   Pescosolido B (1991) Illness careers and network ties: a conceptual model of utilization and compliance. *Advances in Medical Sociology*. **2**: 161–84.

51   Telles J and Pollack M (1981) Feeling sick: the experience and legitimation of illness. *Social Science and Medicine*. **15**(A): 243–51.

52   Rogers A, Popay J, Williams G and Latham M (1997) *Health variations and health behaviour: insights from the qualitative literature*. Health Variations Report I. Health Education Authority, London.

53   Borkan J, Reis S, Hermoni D and Biderman H (1995) Talking about the pain: a patient centred study of low back pain in primary care. *Social Science and Medicine*. **40**: 977–88.

54   Roberts H (1992) Professionals' and parents' perceptions of A&E use in a children's hospital. *Sociological Review*. **40**(1): 109–31.

55   Williams R (1983) Concepts of health: an analysis of lay logic. *Sociology*. **17**(2).

56   Salmon P, Sharma N, Valori R and Bellenger N (1994) Patients' intentions in primary care: relationship to physical and psychological symptoms, and their perception by general practitioners. *Social Science and Medicine*. **38**(4): 585–92.

57   Waitzkin H, Britt T and Williams C (1994) Narratives of ageing and social problems in medical encounters with older persons. *Journal of Health and Social Behaviour*. **35**(4): 322–48.

58   Cartwright A, Hockey L and Anderson J (1973) *Life Before Death*. Routledge, Kegan Paul, London.

59   Tuckett D (1976) *Introduction of Medical Sociology*. Tavistock, London.

60   Gourash N (1978) Help-seeking: a review of the literature. *American Journal of Community Psychology*. **6**(5): 413–23.

61 Shye D, Mullooly J, Freeborn K and Pope C (1995) Gender differences in the relationship between social network support and mortality – a longitudinal study of an elderly cohort. *Social Science and Medicine.* **41**(7): 935–47.

62 Salloway J and Dillon P (1973) A comparison of family networks in health care utilization. *Journal of Comparative Family Services.* **4**: 131–42.

63 Barner M, Evans R, Hertzman C and Lomas J (1982) Ageing and health care utilization: new evidence on old fallacies. *Social Science and Medicine.* **24**(10): 851–62.

64 Calnan N (1983) Social networks and patterns of help-seeking behaviour. *Social Science and Medicine.* **17**: 25–8.

65 Bleeker JK, Lamers LM, Leenders IM, Kruyssen DC *et al.* (1995) Psychological and knowledge factors related to delay of help-seeking by patients with acute myocardial infarction. *Psychotherapy and Psychomatics.* **63**(3–4): 151–8.

66 Scambler G and Scambler A (1984) The illness iceberg and aspects of consulting behaviour. In *The Experience of Illness* (eds R Fitzpatrick *et al.*). Tavistock, London.

67 Pearson M, Dawson C, Moore H and Spence S (1993) Health on borrowed time? Prioritizing and meeting needs in low income households. *Health and Social Care in the Community.* **1**: 11–68.

68 Segall A and Goldstein J (1989) Exploring the correlates of self-provided health care behaviour. *Social Science and Medicine.* **29**(2): 153–61.

69 Dean K (1986) Lay care in illness. *Social Science and Medicine.* **22**(2): 275–84.

70 Segall A (1990) A community survey of self-medication activities. *Medical Care.* **28**(4): 301–10.

71 Dean K (1981) Self-care responses to illness: a selected review. *Social Science and Medicine.* **15**(A): 673.

72 Shuval J, Janetz R and Shye D (1989) Self-care in Israel: physicians' views and perspectives. *Social Science and Medicine.* **29**(2): 233–44.

73 Brown C, Rowley S and Helms P (1994) Symptoms, health and illness behaviour in cystic fibrosis. *Social Science and Medicine.* **39**(3): 375–9.

74   Stoller E, Forster L, Pollow R and Tisdale W (1993) Lay evaluation of symptoms by older people: an assessment of potential risk. *Health Education Q* (United States). **20**(4): 505–22.

75   Dean K (1986) Social support and health: pathways of influence. *Health Promotion*. **1**(2): 133–50.

76   Thompson S, Sobolew-Shubin A, Galbraith M *et al*. (1993) Maintaining perceptions of control: finding perceived control in low-control circumstances. *Journal of Personality and Social Psychology*. **64**(2): 293–304.

77   Blaxter M and Britten N (1996) *Lay Beliefs About Drugs and Medicines and the Implications for Pharmacy Practice*. Pharmacy Practice Research Resource Centre Report, Manchester.

78   Freer C (1980) Self-care: a health diary study. *Medical Care*. **18**: 853.

79   Giachello A, Fleming G and Andersen R (1982) *Self-care Practices in the United States*. Research Project Report. Centre for Health Administration Studies, University of Chicago.

80   Elliott-Binns CP (1986) An analysis of lay medicine: fifteen years later. *Journal of the Royal College of General Practitioners*. **36**: 542–4.

81   Blaxter M and Patterson E (1982) *Mothers and Daughters*. Heinemann, London.

82   Hassell K, Harris J, Rogers A, Noyce P *et al*. (1996) *The Role and Contribution of Pharmacy in Primary Care*. Summary report, NPCRDC, Manchester.

83   Twigg J and Atkins K (1981) *Carers Perceived: Policy and Practice in Informal Care*. Oxford University Press, Oxford.

84   Litwin H (1995) The social networks of elderly immigrants – an analytic typology. *Journal of Ageing Studies*. **9**(2): 155–74.

85   Robinson J (1995) Grief responses, coping processes, and social support of widows. *Nursing Science Quarterly*. **8**(4): 158–64.

86   Thoits PC (1995) Stress, coping and social support processes. Where are we? What next? *Journal of Health and Social Behaviour*. **36** (extra issue): 5, 47–52.

87 Delcadena C, Olavarrieta C and Agudelo Y (1994) Support groups in Mexico for neurologic and psychiatric patients. *Salud Mental.* **17**(4): 7–11.

88 Beam N and Tessaro I (1994) The lay health adviser model in theory and practice – an example of an agency-based programme. *Family and Community Health.* **17**(3): 70–9.

89 Rogers A and Pilgrim D (1991) 'Pulling down churches': accounting for the British mental health users movement. *Sociology of Health and Illness.* **13**(2): 129–48.

90 Hildingh C, Fridlund B and Segesten K (1995) Cardiac nurses' preparedness to use self-help groups as a support strategy. *Journal of Advanced Nursing.* **22**(5): 921–8.

91 van Castern V, Leurquin P, Bartelds A *et al.* (1993) Demand patterns for HIV tests in general practice: information collected by sentinel networks in five European countries. *European Journal of Epidemiology.* **9**(2): 169–75.

92 Pescosolido B and Kroenfeld J (1995) Health illness and healing in an uncertain era: challenges from and for medical sociology. *Journal of Health and Social Behaviour.* **36** (extra issue): 5, 33–46.

93 Hopton J and Dlugolecka M (1995) Need and demand for primary health care: a comparative survey approach. *BMJ.* **310**: 1369–73.

94 George S (1996) *Meeting Demands in Primary Care Services.* Patient Demand Conference, North and Mid Hampshire Health Authority, Winchester. April.

95 Van der Does E and Metz RG (1996) *What Should I Do? Do I Go To The Doctor?* Ketting Partners BV.

96 Gann R (1995) The therapeutic partnership: legal and ethical aspects of consumer health information. *Health Libraries Review.* **12**(2): 83–90.

97 Mahon A (1992) Journey's end. *Health Service Journal.* **102**: 21–2.

98 Paraskevaidis E, Kitchener HC and Walker LG (1993) Doctor–patient communication and subsequent mental health in women with gynaecological cancer. *Psycho-Oncology.* **2**(3): 195–200.

99 Coulter A (1994) Assembling the evidence: patient-focused outcomes research. *Health Libraries Review.* **11**(4): 263–8.

100   Griffiths F (1995) Women's decisions about whether or not to take hormone replacement therapy: influence of social and medical factors. *British Journal of General Practice*. **45**(398): 377–480.

101   Meade CD, McKinney WP and Barnas GP (1994) Educating patients with limited literacy skills: the effectiveness of printed and video-taped materials about colon cancer. *American Journal of Public Health*. **84**(1): 119–21.

102   Wilkin D, Butler T and Coulter A (1997) New models of primary care: developing the future. A development and research programme. *Primary Care Discussion Paper 2*.

103   NHS Executive (1996) *Primary Care: The Future*. NHS Executive, Leeds.

Index